MAX WIQU

STRENGTH TRAINING

The Perfect Guide on How to Achieve That Spartan Physique, Learn The Best Practices, Training and Exercises to Build Your Strength and Have That Spartan Physique You're Dreaming of!

Descrierea CIP a Bibliotecii Naţionale a României
MAX WIQU
   STRENGTH TRAINING. The Ultimate Guide Towards a Happier and Healthier You, Learn All the Useful Information and Tips on How You Can Shape Up and Have a Better Life / Max Wiqu – Bucharest: Editura My Ebook, 2020
   ISBN

MAX WIQU

STRENGTH TRAINING

The Perfect Guide on How to Achieve That Spartan Physique, Learn The Best Practices, Training and Exercises to Build Your Strength and Have That Spartan Physique You're Dreaming of!

My Ebook Publishing House
Bucharest, 2020

TABLE OF CONTENTS

INTRODUCTION

Do we really need to be strong and fit? It depends.

It depends on the type of life we want to lead. Do we want to be "normal"? When normal increasingly means a person who eats junk food all day, abuses their body in every way imaginable and has a body that looks truly terrible in the mirror?

Or do we want to look much better, even beyond normal? Something heroic? Where our bodies are truly a temple that we can be proud of. A body that makes heads turn, feels great and performs how we need to when we need it to.

If you choose the second option, the option of a heroic body, then getting strong and fit is a must.

This Guide gives you a straight path to that goal. Without endless cardio. Without wasting your time on exercises that don't anything. And without the need for expensive supplements, drugs, a personal trainer or any other distractions or potential dangers.

In our Guide you'll approach getting strong and fit with the "take no prisoners" and "accept no excuses" approach of the ancient Spartans. Famous as one of the most strong and fit societies the world has ever produced.

If you've seen any of the "300" movies, or read "Gates of Fire", you'll know exactly why the Spartans are an inspiration. If you haven't see them or read the book, check them out. You'll be glad you did.

Here's some of the things you're about to learn, Spartan style:

The Secrets To Building Powerful Muscle

You've undoubtedly read or been told a ton of misinformation about muscle building. I'm about to share with you secrets that will have you, quickly, becoming stronger and looking better. Without complicated training routines that you'd need a spread sheet to follow.

The Hidden Truth About Recovery

Follow the method in this Guide and you'll never have to worry about "over training" again. The Spartans didn't worry about training too often and you won't either. Nor will you find yourself having to live in the gym.

The Best Way to Lose Fat

Losing fat doesn't have to be complicated, even if you are 100% natural. I'll show you how to get as lean as you'd like to be. All without losing an ounce of muscle, using cardio methods that are both fun and interesting. How to Eat to Build the Body of a Greek God (or Goddess). Yes, you are what you eat. But when you eat can be even more important. The Spartans knew exactly how vital this is to becoming strong and fit and now you will too.

How to Develop the Mind of a Spartan

Once you start thinking like a Spartan, the physique of a Spartan is just a matter of time. Not only will this mindset help you conquer the gym, but it will also enhance every single other area of your life, big and small.

There's more too, of course.

Strong and fit. I'm very happy to have the chance to help you forge the new you, that is overflowing with both these qualities.

Are you ready for battle? Good.

Let's get to work...

CHAPTER 1

STRENGTH TRAINING AS PHYSIQUE BUILDING

If you spend any amount of time inside a mainstream gym, you'll see lots of people pushing around light weights. Not just light weights for you (let's face it everyone has to start somewhere, don't they?), but light weights for THEM.

This isn't how you build a Spartan body.

In fact that's not how you really efficiently build anyone up to being fit, aside from the very few who are blessed with miracle genetics.

We're taking the opposite approach. Perhaps, a harder one, but one which offers quicker and more abundant rewards. We're training to get STRONG.

With strength comes function, health and a fine physique.

A physique that's both "show" and "go."

This is much better than the alternative, trust me.

Breaking Free from the Myths of Bodybuilding

New school bodybuilding brings with it many faulty ideas and methods you are much better doing without. Hopefully, your head isn't too full of them. But in case it is, or even if a few have drifted in, keep these following things in mind while you work through our program and become a Spartan:

High Reps Are A Waste Of Time

Going for a "pump" by performing exercises in endless reps with light weights, a method advocated by many bodybuilding gurus is a waste of time. You're not

"toning" your muscles or whatever else they claim. Instead we will focus on building strength which translates into a better looking body. For most exercises this means staying close to 5 heavy reps.

Stay Away From Too Many Isolation Exercises

Isolation exercises (which are exercises that focus on smaller body parts – things like tricep extensions, calf raises, etc.) have a place, but should NEVER be the main part of a

12

Spartan training program. The over emphasis on these are the reason why many conventional bodybuilding systems fall short.

Avoid Program Ideas That Only Work For People On Drugs

Mainstream bodybuilding magazines are packed with programs that will only work if you are being "chemically" assisted. Our program will get you chiseled and strong without drugs. The Spartans didn't need them. Neither do you.

We're going to work on getting you strong and a great physique too. In this case, you can have your cake and eat it too.

Here's something to keep in mind as we dig into our program:

Take a look at statues of Greek warriors and gods sculpted in the times of the ancients. These images were based on physiques crafted through hard work and smart training, not through strange science or weird modern bodybuilding ideas.

These warriors trained to be STRONG and to be able to FUNCTION WELL on the battlefield. Their appearance was an end result of that training. The same style of training you are also about to embark on.

Combine this with the right style of thinking and the willingness to take action quickly with great resolve and literally anything is possible.

Today can be the birth of a new, strong and powerful you.

I'm betting it is.

CHAPTER 2

WHEN AND WHERE TO TRAIN

To truly develop a Spartan physique and mind-set, training needs to become a priority. This isn't just important as a method of getting fit and strong. It's equally important as a means of ridding yourself of the mental habits and tendencies to be soft and lazy.

So while it's possible to follow abbreviated workout routines and meet some of your physical goals, that's not the path of a Spartan.

Instead we will be training often. The discipline that comes from it is the fire that will burn away the old you and replace it with something better, fitter and stronger!

You will be training five days a week. This 5 day routine will establish the feeling inside that training your body is as much part of your schedule as going to work or school or spending time doing other responsibilities.

It's this type of iron discipline that's possessed by professional athletes and soldiers. It's what separates the men from boys and what will quickly make your dream body a reality.

Each training session will clock in between 45 minutes and one hour, sometimes more depending on the amount and method of cardio.

This will never lead to over training as long as you are getting enough rest and eating a diet that isn't garbage. Both sleep and dietary suggestions are included in this Guide. Follow them and you will never ever have to worry about over training working out five days a week.

Just don't think any of this will be easy. Nothing worthwhile ever is. Just ask the Spartans!

The Question of Where to Train

Most of us have at least a few options of where to train. Let's now consider the most popular and how well they work with our program:

Commercial Fitness Gym

These are the chain gyms filled with people wearing spandex and repping away endlessly on the latest machines while pop music plays in the background. These places are usually the last choice for our Spartan training. While it's still possible to get in a grueling workout while ignoring the atmosphere. If other options are available I suggest you explore them.

Bodybuilder, Powerlifting or CrossFit Gym

Any of these three are much better options. While there programs aren't quite Spartan, you can train seriously in these environments without being distracted by commercial fitness gym nonsense. Just ignore any advice well meaning personal trainers or staff may try to give about your program.

Too many chefs ruin the stew. Follow the ideas in our Guide and see how well they work, rather than mixing things up and possibly not seeing the benefits of training like a Spartan!

Home Gym

If you have a barbell, some dumbbells, a bench and a way to do heavy squats this is a favorite choice of many people who have used this program successfully. You can yell, play loud music, train at whatever time you wish.

The main thing is that friends and family know to not bother you while working out unless it's an absolute emergency.

Five days a week in a place fit for a Spartan to train. Do you think you can handle it?

CHAPTER 3

THE FEW, THE PROUD
(A LOOK AT THE SPARTAN LIFTS)

Building a fit and strong body doesn't require mastering an encyclopedia worth of exercises. The arsenal you'll be using may seem small, but they are all that's necessary.

Experience has shown moving too far away from the list you're about to see is just a distraction. And the last thing you need when getting Spartan fit is too many distractions!

The first three exercises are the real meat of our program. These "big three" have been the basis of the training of practically every supremely fit person you can imagine.

Deadlift Squat Bench Press

Pull Ups / Pull Downs Push Ups

Rows

Shoulder Press Curls

Abdominal Work

There's variations of all these exercises that can "spice" up your training occasionally. But move heavy weights in these lifts (aside for the abdominal work, pull ups and pushups which are more high rep orientated) and you will see an amazing transformation in your body. Fast.

A successful program is all about getting the most out of what you are doing. This is what these crucial exercises provide.

Each of these exercises has their own personalities and tips that we can use to master them more easily. I'll be addressing the most important ones as we dig deeper into our program.

How About Using Machines?

The question about using machines is a natural one. If you believe the fitness industry hype, it's easy to end up thinking that the latest, greatest (and most expensive) machine is the answer to all of your fitness concerns. Now that you're getting caught up to speed on how to train like a Spartan, you've probably guessed this isn't the case.

Using machines over free weights will end up slowing down your progress, limiting your strength and making you more prone to injury. With two exceptions:

1. To Rehab an Injury. If you have sore shoulders and there's no way you can bench press, substituting machine presses on a quality machine is a good option until you are able to bench press again. Shoulder machine presses can also be popular for those with rotator cuff issues. Just use the machines as substitutes until you are able to hit the free weights again. Not a minute longer.

2. To Build up Strength for Full Pull Ups. You'll see pull ups and chin ups are crucial parts of our program. They can be very difficult for those overweight or lacking in upper back and bicep strength. Pull downs on a machine are a way to build up the strength required to train for reps with pull ups and chin ups. The idea is to use heavy pull downs for low reps. Enough of these and you will be able to get the most out of the pull up bar in no time. I'll get into this in more detail in our Spartan pull up chapter.

You should be using free weights and your body weight for resistance at least 90% of the time when you are training. After all, Spartans didn't have Bowflex did they? They didn't need expensive trinkets and you don't either!

CHAPTER 4

HOW THE TRAINING IS STRUCTURED

Here comes our program. Welcome to the ranks of Sparta!

The days we list are suggestions, but suggestions nearly everyone follows. If you work a strange schedule feel free to adjust as needed. Just be sure you are training five days and not doing much too alter the volume of the training. Save these types of alterations, if needed or desired, until you get some experience under your belt.

We'll be training our larger body parts twice a week. One day is reserved for a little extra work for smaller body parts to polish them up a bit. Cardio is also done five days, on every training days.

Monday

Monday will be focused on chest and upper back. Five heavy sets of barbell or dumbbell flat bench presses for five reps each set. These should be done explosively, with a maximum of two minutes rest between each set. Follow these with three sets of push ups. Each set of pushups are done to failure.

After chest move on to either the pull up bar or the pull down machine (if you aren't able to do pull ups). Five sets of pull ups or pull downs. If you are doing pull ups each set is done to failure. If you are working up to pull ups using a pull down machine five sets of five reps.

Again rest two minutes between each set.

After strength training it's on to cardio. No one said this would be easy.

Tuesday

Tuesday you'll be focusing on your ability to pull heavy things off the floor and your legs. Start with five heavy sets of dead lifts for five reps each. Rather than two minutes rest between sets, take three or four minutes as needed.

After dead lifts move on to the squat rack. Barbell squats, five sets of five heavy reps. Two minutes rest between sets. After barbell squats, three sets of body weight squats to failure. Again with two minutes rest between sets.

Follow with cardio.

Wednesday

A rest day. You are going to need it. Especially, when you are getting used to the program. Be sure to get in some good recovery time and try to avoid over-physicality as much as possible. A secret to maximizing recovery is to make sure on rest days to get in a few extra hours of sleep, either at night or in a nap during the day. Added sleep on rest days equals added muscle and better conditioning. When it's time to train, train. When it's time to rest, rest.

Thursday

On Thursday we come back to chest and upper back. Follow the same plan as Monday, but now substitute incline barbell or dumbbell bench presses for flat presses. When you come to pull ups or pull downs reverse your grip, which means you will be doing them chin up style. After back train abs.

Don't forget your cardio.

Friday

Friday, repeat Tuesday's routine. Feel free to substitute a different dead lift or squat version if this appeals to you.

Follow with cardio.

Saturday

Shoulders, biceps and abs are on the menu. A shoulder press of your choice (barbell or dumbbell) of three sets of five reps. Two minutes rest between sets. For biceps do a curl variant of your choice for three sets of five reps. Again with two minutes rest. Finish up with abs and cardio.

Sunday. Rest day. Be sure to write down your plan for the following week.

A busy schedule, but a schedule that produces results without fail. I know you are up for the challenge!

CHAPTER 5

THE SPARTAN DEADLIFT

The dead lift is an exercise that's too often neglected. Which is a huge shame. Not in our Spartan training, where it is one of the three lifts that support our whole program.

To execute a dead lift is simple. But this doesn't mean good form isn't important. Ignore good form on a heavy dead lift and you are asking for injury.

How to Deadlift – Spartan Style

Take a barbell and load it with weights. Have it on the floor a few inches from your feet. Your feet should be slightly more than shoulder width apart. Keep your chest up and your hips down. Squat down to the floor and grab the bar with your hands facing you or, if you prefer, one palm facing you and one palm facing away holding the bar. Be sure to have your head in a neutral position. Pull as you straighten your legs. The bar will stop at mid quad. That's one rep. Lower and repeat.

The dead lift is a brilliant exercise that will pack hard muscle on your entire body as long as you lift HEAVY. We're talking muscle everywhere from your quads to your arms and shoulders. Literally, your entire body. Not many other exercises can make that claim, maybe none other aside from the squat.

These following tips will improve your success with this important lift:

- **Explode Up**. If you pull "slow" you will never develop real power in the dead lift. EXPLODE up. As you become more effective with this lift, you'll find your ability to generate force also expands quickly in your everyday life. This is REAL functional fitness. As an added bonus muscle capable of explosive power looks great too. Many people who were never quite able to get six pack abs start doing heavy dead lifts and end up unveiling them in less than a month.

- **Keep Your Core Tight**. Your abs, lower back and buttocks should all stay tight while you dead lift. This is an important way to protect yourself from injury.

- **NEVER Wear a Weight Lifting Belt**. Not only do weight lifting belts look ridiculous, but they also do more to cause injury than to protect it. They keep your abs and lower back weak. This sustained weakness, while the rest of your torso gets stronger has ended many a weight lifting enthusiast's injury free streak. Never buy a weight lifting belt. If someone gives you one, return it and buy protein powder instead!

Deadlift Variantions Worth Trying

There's two dead lift variations that are a good fit for our program.

Feel free to use either on your second dead lift day of the week if you choose.

- **The Rack Deadlift**. This is done inside a squat rack with the safety bars set at a height equal to your knees, more or less. Place the barbell on the safety bars. This will allow you to lift MUCH heavier since the range of motion is reduced. Otherwise follow the same form as a normal dead lift. Rack dead lifts are excellent for breaking through plateaus in training and building more power.

- **One Armed Deadlift**. You can perform this with either a heavy kettlebell or dumbbell. Focus on speed when you explode up. Be sure to do an equal number of sets with each arm.

If you are ever in a situation where you can only do one exercise, make it the dead lift. It's a Spartan's best friend.

CHAPTER 6

THE SPARTAN SQUAT

Guys with a huge upper body and legs the size of twigs. Go to any mainstream gym and you'll be forced to see this ridiculous sight again and again. Clearly these people aren't training Spartan style. For us, the legs are every bit as important to develop. And they should be for you too.

Powerfully built legs in men and women alike send the not so-subtle message of extreme athleticism. They set you apart from the pack, give you (again) functional strength and are also considered by most to be very attractive.

Are you convinced yet of the need to train legs beyond an occasional set of leg extensions or machine leg presses?

Great. Now let's look at the Spartan Squat.

On the Squat

The squat is an exercise that should never be skipped.

Many people have the temptation to skip it and as a direct result their leg conditioning suffers. Not just leg conditioning, their ENTIRE body conditioning suffers! Heavy squats will pack on muscle in the whole torso. Many old-school bodybuilders and power lifters even preached that the squat was a quick way for men to naturally boost their testosterone levels. Real world results seem to back these ideas up.

Load a heavy barbell either in the squat rack or on squat stands. This is "heavy" for you, but eventually we are aiming for you to build up real power – one and a half times to twice your body weight is a good goal. For now use what you can move for five good reps.

Duck under the bar and rest it on your trapezius. Your feet should be slightly wider than shoulder width apart. Grasp the bar palms facing away from you wherever you find it most comfortable. Most people choose a few inches beyond their shoulders.

Slowly lower yourself to just below parallel. Explode up. This is one rep. Be sure to keep your abs, lower back and glutes tight the entire time you are squatting.

Again, no exercise belts!

Always squat inside a power cage with safety pins or bars set in case a rep is too heavy for you to finish. Or have a partner "spotting" you. Just make sure they are paying close attention! It's no time to be checking email on an iPhone or flirting, that's for sure.

Bodyweight Squats

There's something really special, also, about high rep bodyweight only squats. The warrior cultures of Greece and India swore by them. By using them as a back up to your barbell squats you will be, literally, getting the best leg training method of two worlds (one ancient and one modern) working for you.

Lock your fingers behind your head, elbows pointing to your sides. Position your feet at wider than shoulder width apart. Toes pointing forward. Drop as low as possible. Explode up and repeat for very high reps.

Inhale on the way down and exhale as powerfully as possible on the way up. You'll find body weight squats also build your lung capacity, endurance and fighting spirit in addition to strengthening your legs.

The 300 has legs of steel. Soon you will too!

CHAPTER 7

THE SPARTAN CHEST PRESS

There's little doubt that if most young men were asked what part of their body they'd like to develop powerfully first, the chest would only come in behind the biceps. A large and well defined chest screams strength and fitness.

The Spartan take on the two most common chest presses – the bench press and the pushup gives a quick (but not easy) route to a chest that looks like it's carved from marble. The exercises we focus on may be common, but our approach to them is anything but that.

Follow these instructions and your pectorals will look great and rarely fail you when it comes to function. And nearly anything even remotely athletic depends on a powerful chest. I can't think of one sport that doesn't!

Bench Pressing the Right Way

Now for each of our training sessions where we work the chest press we have a few different options. An honest look in the mirror or once over of your conditioning will determine which choice is best for you. As a default, if you're not sure, turn to the barbell flat bench press.

Barbell Bench Press. This is the bench press almost everyone in the world has tried at least once. You lie flat on a bench, lift a heavy barbell off the bench rack, lower it to the top of your chest and repeat for all of your reps.

Take as wide a grip as comfortable. Touch the chest, but don't slam the bar into it for obvious safety reasons.

Always have safety bars / pins set or use a spotter in case you are unable to make a rep. Explode upwards!

An added old-school safety trick: never use collars to hold the weight plates on the side of the bar. In an extreme emergency you want to be able to slide the weight plates off of the side of the bar. I've been in this situation and, trust me, you'll be glad this is an option with a heavy bar loaded bar across your chest that just won't budge.

Incline Bench Press. The same instructions as the bench press, but with the bench set at an incline. This helps build the upper chest, an area where many people are lacking. I was one of them. After a year of almost exclusive incline bench presses my chest looked it's absolute best.

Dumbbell Press. These can be done in place of either flat or incline bench presses. Less weight is used, but the dumbbells allow for a greater range of motion and are also less harsh on the shoulders. They make for a nice change occasionally.

Spartan Pushups

The pushup is something that is inseparable from the warrior experience. Spartans did them by the hundreds.

So do our modern military units and amateur and professional combat athletes. You will too.

Place your hands slightly more than shoulder width apart. Feet close together. Body in a straight line. Keep your core tight as you explode up. Pushups are done for reps.

Of course there are dozens of pushup variations. As you increase your strength and conditioning feel free to explore them.

Chest training is much more about working hard and smart than it is about following complicated programs. A Spartan chest is within your reach, as long as you take action and grab it!

CHAPTER 8

WARRIOR PULL UPS

The pull up is an exercise that strikes many fitness beginners with complete fear. There's something intimidating, especially if you're on the heavier size, about approaching a pull up bar and finding out you can only do a few reps. Or less.

This shouldn't be intimidating. We all need to start somewhere and we shouldn't be afraid of the truth.

I started off not being able to do more than two or three pull ups. The day I did 25 reps in one set, I felt like superman. Much better than I did the first time I benched my body weight. You will too.

So please be patient when you start doing pull ups if you're not as strong as you'd like to be. Your hard work will be well worth it. And when you grab a pull up bar in a few short months and bang out a set like you were weightless, the reaction of the guys and girls who see you in action will be absolutely priceless.

Getting Started With Pull Ups

When you get started with pull ups low reps (which means however many you can do for each set) are what the game is all about. Even five sets of one or two reps will quickly build your power. If you are unable to do one rep, fall back on low rep sets on a pull down machine until you become strong enough for pull ups. As soon as you can the pull down machine should be abandoned.

How to Perform a Pull Up

Get under a pull up bar. Grab bar with palms facing away from you wider than shoulder width apart. Pull yourself up to the bar as far as possible. Lower yourself and repeat. Through the entire exercise keep your abs and lower body tense. This will help you strengthen your core, while the pull up builds power and size in your entire upper body, especially your back and biceps.

The Difference Between a Pull Up and Chin Up

Chin ups are performed in exactly the same way as pull ups. The only change is that your palms will be facing you rather than away. You'll find the chin adds some nice variety to your workouts. Both are equally effective.

The Power of Negatives

A secret to building pull up and chin up strength and endurance quicker is to work on negatives. After not being able to complete any more reps of either exercise hop up or step up to the "top" position of the exercise and then lower yourself slowly. Repeat for reps. As you build your power in negatives this new strength will carry over into your normal pull ups. Using negatives I've seen women not able to perform two full pull ups build up enough power to do eight within four weeks.

How's that for progress? And don't forget this is quick advances seen from women. Men who have a more favorable bone structure and natural strength can improve even quicker. Give your all to your negative reps!

I hope this has inspired you to put a pull up bar in your house. This is the perfect back up plan for days when it's difficult to make it to the gym.

CHAPTER 9

ABS LIKE A GREEK GOD

When we first think about training the abs and core it's understandable to have the mind flash to the "sexiness" factor of having well defined, visible abs. Nearly every male sex symbol and more than a few female sex symbols have six or eight pack abs. While this is certainly a good reason to carve out "abs of steel" we shouldn't forget the role a strong core has in our ability to function well and also in keeping our body injury free.

So when you train your core like a Spartan you're not only working towards looking like a Greek god (or goddess), but you are also building up your ability to act, injury free like a Spartan warrior.

It doesn't get much better than that.

Hard earned experience has shown that the best way to build a magnificent looking and powerful, functional core is to do a mix of both dynamic and static exercises. Dynamic exercises are when your abs are worked against resistance (often just your own body weight) while static exercises are core and ab exercises when your core is held under tension for short periods of time.

Unlike some of our other body parts variety is a good thing in core training. However, the following exercises are ones you can turn to again and again.

The Crunch

The crunch can be thought of as a more effective version of the old high school favorite, the sit up. Lie on your back with knees bent feet on the floor, hands at the ears. Hold the neck in a neutral position. Curl up the midsection and spine roughly 30 percent towards the knees. Pause, lower back down and repeat. The crunch is done for reps. Three to five sets makes it a foundation of most core training sessions. The crunch can also be done as a "side crunch," with each rep being done towards opposite knees.

Seated Knee Ups

Sitting on a bench or chair grab the seat and lean back slightly. Extend legs in front of you, tensing abs. Pull legs in knees touching abs. Three to five sets done to failure. The knee up trains the lower abs.

Front Plank

Lay on the floor in a push up position, but resting your upper body on your forearms and elbows. Your arms will be in a "L" position elbows in a line with your shoulders. Come up on your toes while tensing core. Hold this position for time, rather then reps. This is an example of a "static" exercise to build your core.

Side Plank

Form a "side pillar" by making a plank but only coming up on one elbow and the side of one foot.

Keep head and neck in a neutral position. Keep core tense for time, over reps. Do an equal number of sets on each side.

Your total core training should consist of 10 sets to failure, split between as many exercises as you choose. Keep the intensity high!

CHAPTER 10

A FEW EXTRA WEAPONS IN THE ARSENAL

Now that we've gone over the major exercises we will be using to build a Spartan warrior-like physique and conditioning, it's on to our assistance exercises. These should be thought of as a kind of "icing on the cake." They are a few extra weapons available in your arsenal. Generally speaking you'll train them one day a week.

They can cover three broad needs we'd like to see filled, which are:

- **They Build up Strength in Weak Areas of the Body.** As perfect as the rest of our program is, the multi-joint exercises do leave a few areas that need to be addressed. These areas are usually smaller body parts, like biceps or shoulders.

- **They Help Increase our Ability to Powerfully Execute our Bigger Lifts.** Sometimes we will hit a plateau in an exercise like the squat or bench press. The missing link to our pushing up more weight can often be worked on with an assistance exercise. Once this weak spot in our muscle chain is focused on and gets caught up to speed our plateau is overcome and we are back to making quick progress!

- **They Help Balance Physiques.** Some of us suffer from slower muscle growth in certain areas. Calves and shoulders are two common examples. If we see this in our own physiques in the mirror, after we have some training under our belts, putting an extra focus on our less developed points can help build a more visually appealing physique.

There's too many potential assistance exercises to list, but here's a few that have proven merit for you when you are following our Spartan program.

Bicep Curls

Who doesn't want large, well-developed biceps?

Bicep curls can be performed with either a barbell or two dumbbells. Some even use exercise bands, which will work too as long as they offer enough reps to keep the exercise range in the 5 rep area.

Pick up the barbell or two dumbbells palms facing away from you. Curl upwards keeping your back straight. Do NOT throw your shoulders back. This is a clear sign of being a person who hits the gym to put on a show, rather than get themselves into top shape!

Shoulder Press

Also gives you the option of using a barbell or dumbbells. This is a TREMENDOUS tool to building shoulders like cannon balls. Don't forget the bigger your shoulders become, the smaller your waist will appear. Makes sense right?

Bring the heavy barbell or dumbbells up to your shoulders. Explode upwards. Only one warning: never do behind the neck presses. They are very, very dangerous and often lead to serious injury.

Shrugs

Shrugs build you're the rear muscles of the shoulders, or traps. Pick up a very heavy barbell palms facing your body. Shrug your shoulders to your ears. Hold for a second. Repeat for reps. Not only will shrugs help you build an athletic looking shoulder and back, but they will also skyrocket your grip strength. Avoid the temptation to use "hand wraps" to reinforce your grip. This is a silly bodybuilder practice that keeps their forearms small and grips weak.

Dips

Feel fortunate if you have a dip station to use. If not perform your dips between two sturdy chairs. Do for high reps. Dips can be thought of as "high octane" push ups and condition the entire upper body. I never skip them on my "day 5" of training where we bang out assistance exercises. Try them and you will likely love them too!

Can you add more assistance exercises to your arsenal? Yes. But don't get too creative until you have some momentum behind you are are more in tune with what your body needs to get the job done!

CHAPTER 11

A DIET TO DIE FOR

An uncomplicated training program that simply works, is best augmented by a diet that is also simple and effective. Spartans don't walk around with little notepads writing down everything they eat as if they were a soccer mom looking to try to lose twenty summer pounds.

Instead, we follow broad principles. Broad principles which will help build muscle and burn fat.

Keep these things in mind concerning diet. Remember, without some diet discipline there's no way you will ever be able to build a body to die for. Take action on these points and a body worthy of "300" can be yours as long as your training and lifestyle are in order.

Small Fasts Every Day

The first, and most important part of your Spartan diet is that you will only be eating twice a day. Yes, twice a day.

A lunch at roughly 1 or 2pm (depending on your schedule) and a large dinner at 6 or 7. No snacking, no food after dinner and no breakfast.

You may notice this is nearly the same as some forms of "intermittent fasting." It certainly is. In fact, Spartans were among the first intermittent fasters. There's no better way to lose fat while building muscle. And there's no better way to build a warrior mind-set.

Is it hard at first? Yes. But you can and should do it. Your body will thank you by looking its best.

No Drinking Calories

Drinking empty calories is something that keeps people fat. Substitute water, green tea, coffee or, even, diet drinks (if you must). Many of my clients have found this one simple diet alteration sped up their amount of fat- loss by over ten pounds a month! Be disciplined and stop drinking calories immediately.

Eat Clean Protein With Every Meal

Protein is the building block of muscle. You should not only be eating it with every meal, but take every effort to eat as lean a form of protein as possible. Choose fish and chicken over fatty cuts of beef and pork whenever possible.

Vegetables are Your Friend

Eat a wide range of vegetables. The less you cook them the better. It's basically impossible to over eat vegetables and they are fantastic for fighting hunger pains. They will also help you detoxify and stay detoxified.

Don't Overeat Carbohydrates

Yes, you need carbs when you are following as active a program as a Spartan.

This doesn't mean to go crazy overeating carbs. Most fat people are carb addicts. Fight the temptation and lean towards protein and vegetables whenever and wherever you can. Rice, some potatoes, beans and fruit are acceptable. Processed carbs cooked up in a laboratory are absolutely not!

Read Labels

As a new master of your destiny you are completely responsible for what you put into your body. This means taking the time to read and understand what you are eating and drinking. Being a warrior is being an independent thinker. Don't let sneaky marketing entice you into buying things you don't need as they get rich.

There you go. A diet strategy that won't ever let you down, as long as you train hard and keep your mind in the game. Stop making excuses and start eating like a Spartan!

CHAPTER 12

THINKING LIKE THE 300

The best plans or program will never work for you until you have a mind that is disciplined enough to follow it. Spartan warriors were known for having developed a mind-set that addressed the problems that came along with dedication to a strict training and the "religion" of physical culture. You can learn to think like the 300 too. Once you do, you are at least half way towards having the body of your dreams.

When it comes to thinking like a proud member of the 300 remember these things:

Think Positively

The mind can be something that drains you or motivates you when you face challenges. And getting into great shape is certainly a tough challenge for many of us.

Adopting the habit of thinking and speaking positively has absolutely nothing to do with "new age" mysticism. It has everything to do with being able to perform optimally. Clear your mind of negative self-talk and immediately replace it with "can do" messages. Watch how much more power this will give you to get things done almost instantly!

Be Prepared for Sacrifice

Nothing really exceptional good can happen without hard work. That's a truth that is unavoidable despite what the mainstream supplement hawkers and "fitness professionals" may try to sell you. If you want to be everything you can be you MUST be prepared to work hard. Chiseling out a new body isn't easy, but the method in this Guide will make it EASIER than it could be. All your sweat, time and hard work will be worth it. Trust me.

Write Down Your Goals

Spartans are goal setters and achievers.

Taking a few minutes a day to write down your daily goals and a half hour or so on the weekend to work out weekly and monthly goals can be the difference between being successful with your program and failing. All winners are goal setters.

Historical studies have even shown that the Spartan leaders were near obsessive about their planning, much more so than any other leaders of their time. Once you have a target it is much easier to accomplish it!

The Willingness to Take Action

This is the most important Spartan mental trait you should adopt if you want to accomplish your physical aspirations. Embracing this mind-set will also make accomplishing ANYTHING much easier.

It's what 95% of the people in the world are lacking. The willingness to take quick action. You can have all the knowledge in the world and the best of intentions, but if you don't act on them the chances of change occurring in your life is cut down to almost nothing. Act quickly and often and you at least have a fighting chance of seeing your life improve. Sitting around and feeling sorry for yourself will get you nowhere – fast!

There it is. Training methods and winning attitudes that worked in the past will work just as well today. We are still the same human beings with the same physical make-ups that respond the same way to adversity.

Adopting our unique Spartan approach will quickly send weakness on the run. Are you ready to join the 300? Then get up and start working hard today!

BONUS FAQ

Question: I really like the training program, but is it possible to get good results while following a different diet plan? I want to get Spartan fit, but I find it really difficult to follow the intermittent fasting style protocol.

Answer: You can pick whichever parts of our Guide most appeal to you and use them. It's better than doing nothing. But I'd suggest giving the program a shot as a whole and seeing your results. Don't forget it's often the things we like the least, that help us the most! A personal example is that I'd hated squats for years. And I had skinny legs. I made every excuse not to squat and my legs never really grew. One day I committed to squatting for thirty days and seeing if it made a difference. It did. Now my legs are one of my more appealing body parts and I've learned to love squatting. Try our diet plan and you may end up feeling the same way!

Question: What type of cardio should I be doing?

Answer: Anything that get's your hard beating hard and your body sweating. Investigate HIIT cardio (high intensity interval training) and you can really get the most out of a short session. Don't neglect sports either, especially boxing and martial arts. These are all methods that worked to help keep the Spartan warrior fit and lean and they will you to. Plus you won't die of boredom in the process.

Question: The tone of your Guide is "man" orientated. Will this program work for a woman too? My girlfriend would like to join me in training.

Answer: Yes, 100%. There's only slight changes I suggest for most women. For chest training sessions most women should focus on incline presses over flat presses, for example. Building a well developed upper chest and shoulders ends up with a more flattering end result for most women who train, rather than working on the "middle chest" with flat presses. Otherwise, there's not much of a need to adjust many things. Women are more than welcome to join us in the 300!

Question: I was surprised you don't really mention supplements at all. Do you have any supplement suggestions?

Answer: Supplements are really a personal decision. Most, beyond fish oil, a multi vitamin, protein shakes and creatine are a waste of time and money. It's much better to devote your time and energy to training, diet and rest than chasing the latest "miracle in a bottle." Believe me, if these things existed you wouldn't see so many fat people everywhere you turn.

Question: I really like training on machines at my gym. Your Guide really seems to discourage using them too often. Aren't they putting the latest technology towards the goal of building better bodies?

Answer: Simply stated, no. Train on a bench press machine for six months and an average guy may be about to lift two hundred and fifty pounds or more. Take that same guy and ask him to bench press a barbell and don't be shocked if he can't do one rep with 185lbs. I've seen it dozens of times. Take the same guy and see if he can help you move furniture or something similar. You're likely to, again, be disappointed.

Machines may make a person look bigger and they may build "numbers" on that machine, but this isn't power that carries over into real life. Our goal is to get you strong and fit. Not help you build cosmetic muscles with no practical use at all! Let the machines collect dust. Pick up some heavy weights!

Good luck and thanks for reading!

Printed by Libri Plureos GmbH in Hamburg, Germany